Diabetic Renal Diet Cookbook For Newly Diagnosed

A Complete Diabetes and Kidney Health Recipe

Mclan O. Micheals, RDN

Disclaimer

The information provided in this guide is for educational purposes only and should not replace professional medical advice. Before making any big dietary changes, remember to speak with a medical practitioner or a certified dietitian to be sure they are in line with your unique medical requirements.

Copyright © 2023, Mclan O. Micheals, RDN

All rights reserved.

Diabetic Renal Diet Cookbook For Newly
Diagnosed

Table of Contents

Diabetic Renal Diet Cookbook For Newly Diagnosed

Diabetic Renal Diet Cookbook For Newly Diagnosed

Introduction

This book is intended to help those who are navigating the difficult road of controlling diabetes and renal health by offering critical advice, support, and delectable recipes.

Millions of individuals throughout the globe suffer from a complicated disease known as diabetes. Diet, medicine, exercise, and lifestyle decisions need to be carefully considered. Managing these illnesses may be very difficult when renal issues are present. However, it is possible to live a satisfying life while successfully managing diabetes and renal health provided you have the correct information, resources, and a good outlook.

Please allow me to tell you about Sonia, a young lady in her forties who is vivacious and active. Sonia received the news that she had diabetes a few years ago, which shocked her. She started a path of education about the condition, essential lifestyle adjustments, and vigilant blood sugar monitoring. She was adamant about leading a balanced life despite the difficulties.

But when Sonia began to have renal issues, her journey took an unexpected turn. Her everyday activities became much more complicated once she was diagnosed with renal problems. She was bewildered by the complicated connections between diabetes and renal function and was unclear about how to proceed. She found herself in need of clear direction, useful counsel, and, most crucially, delectable dishes that would support her dual health objectives, just like many others confronting similar circumstances.

Sonia's experience is not unusual. Renal problems and newly diagnosed diabetics may present comparable difficulties. Our goal is to provide you with the information, tactics, and culinary inspiration you need to properly manage your health.

This cookbook has a wealth of knowledge, delicious recipes, and helpful advice that is created especially for those with diabetes and kidney issues. You will get thorough instructions on how to comprehend diabetes and kidney health, the fundamentals of the diabetic renal diet, nutritional recommendations, meal planning advice, cooking methods, and much more in each chapter.

But there's more to this book than simply numbers and statistics. It involves adopting a constructive and proactive attitude toward your health. It is about enjoying the process of preparing delicious meals that are also nutritious. It involves accepting responsibility

for your health and embracing the opportunities
that lie ahead.

So this book is here to be your companion on
this path, whether you are a newly diagnosed
person searching for clarity and support or a
caregiver wanting to prepare nourishing and
delectable meals for your loved ones. We'll
delve into the realm of diabetic renal cuisine
together, learn about the benefits of wholesome
foods, and set off on a journey to greater health
and well-being.

Let's start this life-changing journey one meal at
a time as we embark on a culinary journey that
honors the balance between the management of
diabetes and renal health.

Keep in mind that you are not alone. You have
the resources, information, and encouragement
you need to adopt a diabetic renal diet and

enjoy a full, active life if you have this

cookbook in your possession. Let's get going!

Diabetic Renal Diet Cookbook For Newly Diagnosed

Mclan O.Micheals, RDN   11

Chapter One

Understanding Diabetes and Kidney Health

Type 1 and type 2 diabetes often develop major
consequences called diabetic nephropathy,
which is also called diabetic renal disease. By
leading a healthy lifestyle and effectively
treating your diabetes and high blood pressure,
you may stop or postpone diabetic nephropathy.

The disorder gradually weakens the sensitive
filtration mechanism in your kidneys over many
years. Early diagnosis and treatment may lessen
the likelihood of complications and stop or
decrease the disease's progression.

Renal failure, often known as end-stage kidney
disease, may result from renal disease. A
life-threatening ailment, kidney failure. Dialysis

or a kidney transplant are the only available
treatments at this time.

Symptoms

You would probably not have any symptoms or
indicators in the early stages of diabetic
nephropathy. You could see these signs later:

- Deteriorating blood pressure regulation
- Urine contains protein.
- Swelling of the hands, eyes, feet, or
  ankles
- Increased urination frequency
- Less insulin or diabetic medication is
  required
- Confusion or attentional issues
- Breathing difficulty
- Reduced appetite
- Nausea and diarrhea
- Chronic itching
- Fatigue

When It Becomes Mandatory to See a Doctor

If you have any indications that you may have kidney disease, schedule an appointment with your doctor. If you have diabetes, you should have kidney function tests performed at least once a year or as otherwise advised by your doctor.

Diabetic Renal Diet Cookbook For Newly Diagnosed

Chapter Two

Essential Nutrients for Diabetic Renal Health

For those with type 2 diabetes who also have kidney disease as a consequence of their illness, diet is a crucial part of treating the disease. This is because extra nutrients, poisons, and fluids may build up in the blood when the kidneys aren't operating regularly.

The majority of patients with severe kidney disease are referred to a renal dietitian, a nutritionist who focuses on kidney illness since it is such a serious issue. A tailored eating strategy may be created by this expert that takes your medical history, treatment objectives, and current health into consideration.

Maintaining a healthy diet while adhering to dietary limitations that promote kidney function in people with diabetes may be challenging. For instance, some essential nutrients should be avoided, yet they occasionally appear in unexpected meals. Others are available in various forms (like fat) so attention should be used while selecting them.

Sodium

A crucial component in the fluids that envelop cells is sodium. Together with potassium, it controls the body's fluid balance and blood pressure. It is essential for the healthy operation of the muscles and neurological system and aids in maintaining PH equilibrium.

Why Kidney Disease Matters

Sodium may build up in cells and cause fluid to collect in tissues when the kidneys begin to fail, resulting in swelling known as edema. Lower extremities, hands, and the face are often affected by edema.

Additionally, too much salt raises blood pressure (hypertension), results in breathlessness, and creates fluid around the heart and lungs. An excessive amount of salt in the diet may worsen edema and harm the kidneys.

Your body retains a lot of fluid and salt when your kidneys are unhealthy. Ankle swelling, puffiness, an increase in blood pressure, shortness of breath, and/or fluid around your heart and lungs may all result from this.

Suggested Intake

The Centers for Disease Control and Prevention (CDC) estimate that around 3,400 milligrams (mg) of salt are consumed daily by most Americans, which is more than is advised. Less than 2,300 mg per day is advised by the Dietary Guidelines for Americans.3

Normally, it is suggested that those with chronic kidney disease (CKD) take considerably less salt.

Table salt naturally contains sodium, so using it sparingly may help reduce sodium consumption. But a large range of foods also includes salt. Only 10% of the salt that Americans eat is, according to the National Kidney Foundation (NKF), eaten at home (in cooking and at the table). The remaining food is obtained from supermarkets and restaurants.

Knowing where salt may be hiding is crucial if you're on a low-sodium diet to treat diabetes and/or renal disease so that you can limit your consumption within the ranges advised by your doctor or nutritionist.

Potassium

The majority of bodily processes, such as kidney and heart function, muscular contraction, and nervous system message transmission, all need potassium.

Why Kidney Disease Matters

Although potassium is crucial for kidney health, an excess of it in the blood, known as hyperkalemia, may be dangerous. When the kidneys are sick, this may occur.

A potassium overdose may be risky since it can result in an irregular cardiac rhythm, which can then go bad enough to trigger a heart attack.

If you have a renal illness, your doctor will likely do monthly blood tests to check your potassium levels and make sure they haven't risen to dangerous levels.

Suggested Intake

The Office of Dietary Supplements, a division of the National Institutes of Health (NIH), recommends that adult males (19 years of age and older) consume 3,400 mg of potassium per day. 2,600 mg should be consumed by adult women.

Potassium is included in a broad range of foods, making it very simple to consume enough quantities of it daily.

However, due to its accessibility, those who have diabetes, renal disease, or both should be aware of the foods that are the highest sources of potassium so they may control their consumption.

Phosphorus

Although it is present in tiny quantities in DNA, cell membranes, and teeth, phosphorus is a mineral that is mostly retained in bones.

It is important for numerous bodily functions and responses, including the conversion of food into energy, muscular contraction, nerve transmission, and normal kidney function. Strong bones are also aided by phosphorus.

Why Kidney Disease Matters

When in good health and operating correctly, the kidneys remove extra phosphorus from the blood. This process is hampered by renal illness, and phosphorus may build up.

Bones become weaker as a result of too much phosphorus removing calcium from them. Aside from that, excessive amounts of phosphorus and calcium may cause calcium deposits in the lungs, eyes, heart, and blood vessels, which over time can raise the risk of heart attack, stroke, and death.

Phosphorus is problematic because, even when blood levels rise severely, a condition known as hyperphosphatemia, there are no obvious signs. Typically, stage 4 chronic renal disease is needed for the syndrome to become apparent.

Suggested Intake

Dietary Guidelines for Americans state that those aged 19 and older should consume 700 mg of phosphorus daily.

Several different foods and drinks contain phosphorus, especially:

Ale and beer, chocolate and cocoa beverages, dark colas and sodas, Iced tea in a can, dairy items such as milk, milk-based beverages, cheese, custard and pudding, ice cream, and soups made with cream are also included. Oysters, sardines, salmon roe, organ meats such as beef liver, chicken liver, and others; a chocolate treat, caramels, muffins with oat bran, alcoholic yeast, fast food, prepared meals, canned and bottled beverages, boosted meats, and the majority of processed foods often include phosphorus. Look for the letters "phos" on the ingredient list to prevent phosphorus additions.

Carbohydrates

The body uses nutrients called carbohydrates as its main source of energy. Simple carbohydrates, which are essentially sugars, provide energy very quickly after eating, and complex carbohydrates, often known as starches, are changed into glycogen, which is then stored and utilized as a fuel in the future. Any extra carbs have the potential to turn into fat.

Why It Matters for Kidney Disease

Managing diabetes is crucial for repairing the renal damage it has caused.

This is because one of the factors contributing to kidney damage brought on by diabetes is high blood sugar (glucose) levels.

Recommended Intake

Approximately half of the daily calories should come from carbs, according to the Dietary Guidelines for Americans, but it's not quite that straightforward. For instance, complex carbohydrates are better for you than simple ones. Age, weight, height, and degree of exercise are further factors.

Ideal carbohydrate consumption for adults with diabetes also relies on daily blood glucose levels, especially for those who use insulin to treat their condition.

It is neither wise nor essential to completely cut out carbs from your diet if you have diabetes-related renal damage.

But you need to be very selective about the kinds of carbohydrates you consume. To stay on the safe side, avoid simple carbohydrates and consume just the recommended quantity of complex carbohydrates. You may want to reduce your consumption of carbohydrates that are high in potassium and/or phosphorus.

Protein

Amino acids, which are smaller molecules, are used to build protein molecules. When protein-rich meals are consumed, the body disassembles them and then reassembles the amino acids to produce the protein structures it requires. Protein is used by the human body for almost everything.

Protein is a component of hemoglobin, skin, hair, muscles, and other tissues. Proteins also serve as building blocks for enzymes, which

metabolize food and start chemical processes.
Additionally, a lot of hormones, such as insulin
and other hormones that control metabolism,
are proteins.

Protein is necessary for the immune system to
produce antibodies. The exchange of signals
between neurotransmitters in the brain is also
facilitated by protein molecules.

Why Kidney Disease Is Important

Kidney damage may prevent a person from
getting rid of all the waste that is produced
when they take protein. The kidneys may
experience detrimental wear and tear as a result
of having to cope with more of this waste.

A buildup of protein waste may result in
symptoms including nausea, lack of appetite,
weakness, and changes in how foods taste, in

addition to additional harm to already weakened kidneys.

Suggested Intake

The amount of protein that should be consumed daily is 0.8 grams for every kilogram of body weight. That amounts to 0.36 grams per pound, which is under 10% of your daily caloric intake.

Your daily recommended protein intake is calculated by multiplying your weight by 0.36. If you weigh 150 pounds, for instance, the recommended daily intake of protein is 54 grams (unless you engage in physical activity, in which case it should be more).

Reducing protein consumption may help people with CKD decrease the disease's development, according to studies. There aren't any set rules for cutting protein, however.

Several personal considerations, including whether or not someone is receiving dialysis, will determine how large a reduction a person should make.

All of the necessary amino acids are present in animal proteins, although certain sources, such as fatty cuts of red meat, whole-milk dairy products, and egg yolks, may include a lot of harmful (saturated) lipids.

Fish, poultry, and low-fat or fat-free dairy products are preferable options for everyone, not only those with CKD or other illnesses or disorders since they contain the fewest saturated fats.

Beans, lentils, nuts, peanut butter, seeds, and whole grains are examples of plant sources of protein. These often lack one or more essential amino acids, but when eating a well-planned plant-based or vegetarian diet, it is feasible to receive all the necessary ones. Additionally advantageous are plant proteins' low saturated fat and high fiber content.

Overall health is critically dependent on healthy fats. The National Institute of Diabetes and Digestive and Kidney Disease (NIDDKD) states that it helps control blood pressure and other cardiac functions, provides energy, is a component of membranes throughout the body, transports vital fat-soluble vitamins A, D, E, and K, and contains carotenoids.

Why Kidney Disease Is Important

There are certain harmful fats. Persons with CKD who are already more vulnerable to these issues than the majority of people may have elevated blood cholesterol and blocked blood vessels, raising the risk of a heart attack or stroke.

Suggested Intake

No more than 25% to 35% of the daily calories that the majority of individuals in the general population should get from dietary fats. Saturated fat should make up no more than 7% of daily calories. Most individuals should try to keep their daily cholesterol consumption to around 300 mg.

For people with chronic renal disease and the medical experts who care for them, figuring out how much fat to include in their diets may be a delicate balancing act. It involves being aware of the bad fats and avoiding them as much as you can while making sure you get enough beneficial fats without consuming too many calories.

Chapter Three

Breakfast and Brunch Recipes

Veggie Omelet

Ingredients:

2 eggs

Diced bell peppers, chopped onions, 1/4 cup

1/4 cup diced tomatoes

1/4 cup chopped spinach

Pepper and salt to taste

Method:

- Coat the pan with cooking oil or nonstick cooking spray.

- Beat the eggs thoroughly in a basin.

- Before heating a non-stick pan, it should be lightly coated with cooking spray or olive oil.

- Bell peppers and onions, diced, should
  be added to the pan and cooked for a few
  minutes until tender.
- Diced tomatoes and chopped spinach
  should be added to the pan and cooked
  for another minute.
- The eggs that have been beaten should
  be poured over the vegetables in the pan.
- After a few minutes of cooking, the
  edges of the omelet should start to firm
  up.
- After gently folding the omelet in half,
  cook it for another minute until the eggs
  are thoroughly cooked.
- Add pepper and salt to taste.
- Eat the hot veggie omelet right away.

Greek yogurt parfait

Ingredients:

Plain Greek yogurt in 1/2 cup

1/4 cup of fresh berries, such as strawberries,

blueberries, or raspberries

1 tablespoon of nuts, such as almonds or

walnuts, that have been coarsely chopped

One optional spoonful of honey Technique:

Method:

- Place Greek yogurt, fresh fruit, and
  coarsely chopped almonds in a bowl or
  glass.
- Add a honey drizzle, if desired.
- Repeat the layers if desired.
- The parfait with Greek yogurt needs to
  be chilled.

Quinoa Breakfast Bowl

Ingredients:

1/2 cup of cooked quinoa

Slices of almonds in 1/4 cup

Fresh fruits, such as apples, pears, or bananas,

cut into 1/4 cup

1 tbsp. chia seeds

1 tablespoon honey or maple syrup (optional)

an optional sprinkle of cinnamon

Method:

- On a plate, combine the cooked quinoa, almond pieces, fruit cubes, and chia seeds.

- Sprinkle honey or maple syrup, if preferred.

- Add a little cinnamon powder if you'd like.

- Stir well to completely combine all ingredients.

- You may either serve the quinoa breakfast meal cold or at room temperature.

Whole-grain Pancakes

Ingredients:

1 cup whole wheat flour

Baking soda, 1 teaspoon

1 tablespoon of honey or maple syrup

One cup of nonfat milk

1 large egg, with the pan coated with olive oil
or frying spray.

Method:

- Add whole wheat flour and baking powder to a bowl.
- Combine the low-fat milk, egg, and honey or maple syrup in a separate bowl.
- The dry ingredients must be combined with the liquid ones while swirling constantly to create a homogenous batter.
- Before heating a nonstick pan or griddle, lightly grease it with cooking spray or olive oil.
- 1/4 cup of the batter should be added to the skillet for each pancake.
- Cook until surface bubbles emerge, then flip the food over and cook for an

additional minute, or until golden brown
on both sides.

- Use the leftover batter to continue.
- If desired, drizzle some honey or maple
syrup on top of the heated whole-grain
pancakes.

Toast with Egg and Avocado

Ingredients:

1 slice of whole-grain bread

A mashed avocado, half-ripe

1 fried or poached egg with preferred amounts
of pepper and salt

Method:

- Toast the whole-grain bread till golden
brown.
- Distribute the mashed avocado in an
even layer on the toasty bread piece.
- On top, place a cooked or poached egg.
- Add pepper and salt to taste.

- It is best to serve the avocado toast with eggs immediately.

Frittata with Mushrooms and Spinach

Ingredients:

4 eggs

Half a cup of spinach, chopped

Using olive oil or cooking spray to coat the pan, add the chopped mushrooms

1/4 cup sliced onions

Pepper and salt as desired

Method:

- Beat the eggs thoroughly in a basin.
- Before heating a non-stick pan, it should be lightly coated with cooking spray or olive oil.
- Sliced mushrooms, diced onions, and chopped spinach should all be added to the pan. Sauté the veggies for a few minutes, or until they start to soften.

- The beaten eggs should be poured over the vegetables in the pan.

- Cook the frittata for a few minutes, or until the edges start to set.

- Place the pan on a hot broiler for a few minutes, or until the top is done and just starting to brown.

- Add salt and pepper to taste.

- Cut the frittata into wedges.

- You may choose to serve the spinach and mushroom frittata hot or cold.

Enjoy these breakfast and brunch recipes for the health of your diabetic kidneys as part of a balanced diet, and feel free to change the ingredients and serving sizes to fit your preferences and dietary needs.

Chapter Four

Satisfying Lunch and Dinner Recipes

Grilled Chicken with Lemon, Herbs, and Roasted Vegetables

Ingredients:

4 chicken breasts, skinless and boneless

Lemon juice, two teaspoons

Olive oil, 1 tbsp

1 teaspoon dry herbs, such as rosemary, oregano, or thyme

Pepper and salt as desired

2 cups of roasted veggies, including onions, bell peppers, and zucchini

Method:

- Lemon juice, olive oil, dried herbs, salt, and pepper should all be combined in a dish.

- Put the chicken breasts in the marinade and let them at least 30 minutes to marinate.

- Set the grill's temperature to medium-high.

- The chicken breasts should be cooked through and no longer pink in the middle after grilling for 6 to 8 minutes on each side.

- Roast the mixed veggies in a preheated oven at 400°F (200°C) for approximately 20 minutes, or until they are soft, while the chicken is cooking.

- Serve the roasted veggies beside the grilled chicken with lemon and herbs.

Broccoli and Quinoa with Baked Salmon

Ingredients:

2 filets of salmon

One teaspoon of lemon juice

Olive oil, 1 tbsp

One tablespoon of dried dill

Pepper and salt as desired

Cooked quinoa, 1 cup

Florets of steam-cooked broccoli

Method:

- Set the oven's temperature to 400°F (200°C).
- Put the Salmon fillets on a baking pan covered with parchment paper.
- Olive oil and lemon juice should be drizzled over the fish.
- Over the fish, season with salt and pepper and dried dill.

- The salmon should be baked for 12 to 15 minutes, or until it is cooked through and flakes readily.

- Serve the baked salmon with steamed broccoli and cooked quinoa.

Stir-fried Turkey and Vegetables

Ingredients:

Olive oil, 1 tbsp

1/2 pound of ground turkey

1 cup of sliced mixed veggies, including carrots, snap peas, and bell peppers

2 minced garlic cloves

Low-sodium soy sauce, 1 tbsp

1 teaspoon optional sesame oil

Pepper and salt as desired

Brown rice or whole wheat noodles that have been cooked

Method:

- In a skillet or wok, warm the olive oil over medium heat.
- Cook the ground turkey in the pan until it is well-cooked and browned.
- Stir-fry the sliced mixed veggies for a few minutes, or until they are tender-crisp, in the pan with the minced garlic.
- Add the sesame oil (if using) and low-sodium soy sauce.
- Add salt and pepper to taste.
- Serve the stir-fried turkey and vegetables on their own or, if preferred, with cooked brown rice or whole wheat noodles.

Vegetable and Lentil Soup

Ingredients:

1 cup of washed and drained dry lentils

Olive oil, 1 tbsp

1 chopped onion, 2 diced carrots, 2 diced celery

stalks, and 2 minced garlic cloves

Low salt vegetable broth, 4 cups

2-cups of water

One tablespoon of dried thyme

Bay leaf, one

Pepper and salt as desired

Method:

- Warm the olive oil in a big saucepan, on
  a medium heat.
- When the veggies begin to soften, add
  the minced garlic, diced carrots, diced
  celery, and chopped onion to the
  saucepan.
- To the saucepan, add the washed lentils,
  water, vegetable broth, dried thyme, and
  bay leaf.
- The soup should be brought to a boil,
  then simmered for 25 to 30 minutes, or
  until the lentils are soft.

- Add pepper and salt to taste.
- Before serving, take the bay leaf out.
- Serve the hot vegetable and lentil soup.

Quinoa salad with Grilled Lemon Herb Shrimp Skewers

Ingredients:

1 pound of peeled and deveined shrimp

Lemon juice, two teaspoons

Olive oil, 1 tbsp

1 teaspoon of dry herbs, such as thyme, basil, or parsley

pepper and salt as desired

Cooked quinoa

Cucumbers, tomatoes, and red onions cut into dice

Chopped fresh herbs, like mint or parsley

Serving slices of lemon

Method:

- Lemon juice, olive oil, dried herbs, salt, and pepper should all be combined in a dish.

- For approximately 15 minutes, add the shrimp to the marinade and let them soak.

- Set the grill's temperature to medium-high.

- The marinated shrimp are threaded onto skewers.

- The shrimp skewers should be cooked through and opaque after 2 to 3 minutes on each side of the grill.

- Combine the cooked quinoa with the diced cucumbers, tomatoes, red onions, and fresh herbs in a separate dish.

- Add salt, pepper, lemon juice, and olive oil to the quinoa salad.

- Along with the quinoa salad and lemon
  wedges, serve the grilled lemon herb
  shrimp skewers.

Baked Chicken and Veggie Casserole

Ingredients:

4 skinless, boneless breasts of chicken

2 cups of chopped mixed veggies, such as

carrots, broccoli, and cauliflower

1 cup of chicken broth low in salt

Olive oil, two teaspoons

2 minced garlic cloves

1 teaspoon dried herbs, like thyme, rosemary, or

oregano

Pepper and salt as desired

Method:

- Set the oven's temperature to 375°F
  (190°C).
- Place the chicken breasts and the
  chopped mixed veggies in a baking dish.

- Combine the chicken broth, olive oil, minced garlic, dried herbs, salt, and pepper in a separate bowl.

- Over the chicken and veggies in the baking dish, pour the mixture.

- When the chicken is cooked through and the veggies are soft, cover the baking dish with foil and bake for approximately 25 to 30 minutes.

- To allow the chicken to gently brown during the last 10 minutes of baking, remove the foil.

- The hot chicken and vegetable dish should be served.

- Enjoy these lunch and supper dishes for diabetic renal health as a part of your calorie-controlled diet. Keep in mind to modify the ingredients and serving quantities to suit your own dietary requirements and tastes.

Chapter Five

Healthy Snacks and Appetizers

Yogurt and Cucumber Dip

Ingredients:

1 peeled and grated cucumber

1 cup of Greek yogurt, plain

2 minced garlic cloves

One teaspoon of lemon juice

1 tablespoon freshly chopped dill

Pepper and salt as desired

Method:

- Apply a clean kitchen towel to the shredded cucumber and squeeze out any extra moisture.

- Grated cucumber, Greek yogurt, minced garlic, lemon juice, and chopped dill should all be combined in a dish.

- Add pepper and salt to taste.

- All components should be well mixed.

- Serve cold with carrot, celery, or bell pepper sticks made from fresh vegetables.

Baked Sweet Potato Fries

Ingredients:

Two little sweet potatoes

Olive oil, 1 tbsp

1 paprika teaspoon

1/2 tsp. of garlic powder

Pepper and salt as desired

Method:

- A baking sheet should be lined with parchment paper and the oven should be preheated to 425°F (220°C).

- Cut the sweet potatoes into thin fries after peeling them.

- Sweet potato fries should be mixed with olive oil, paprika, garlic powder, salt, and pepper in a bowl.
- On the baking sheet that has been prepared, spread the fries in a single layer.
- Fries should be baked for 20 to 25 minutes, turning once halfway through, until crispy and golden brown.
- Serve hot as a wholesome and low-sodium substitute for regular French fries.

Chickpeas Roasted

Ingredients:

1 can of drained and washed chickpeas

Olive oil, 1 tbsp

1 paprika teaspoon

1/2 tsp. cumin

1/2 tsp. of garlic powder

Salt as desired

Method:

- A baking sheet should be lined with parchment paper and the oven should be preheated to 400°F (200°C).

- To eliminate extra moisture, pat dry the washed chickpeas with a paper towel.

- Chickpeas should be mixed with salt, olive oil, paprika, cumin, and garlic powder in a bowl.

- On the prepared baking sheet, distribute the chickpeas in a single layer.

- Roast the chickpeas until they are crisp and brown, approximately 30-35 minutes, stirring the pan now and again.

- Before serving the roasted chickpeas as a protein- and fiber-rich snack, let them cool.

Caprese Skewers

Ingredients:

Plum tomatoes

Balls of fresh mozzarella

Fresh leaves of basil

Balsamic glaze, if desired

Method:

- On a skewer, arrange a cherry tomato, a ball of fresh mozzarella, and a basil leaf.
- Until you have the required number of skewers, repeat the procedure.
- If used, drizzle with balsamic glaze.
- Serve as a light appetizer or snack choice that is low in carbohydrates.

Greek Salad Stuffed Cucumbers

Ingredients:

2 substantial cukes

Diced tomatoes, 1 cup

1 cup of cucumbers, diced

1/2 cup red onion, chopped

1/2 cup feta cheese crumbles

2 teaspoons freshly chopped parsley

Lemon juice, two teaspoons

Extra virgin olive oil, 1 tablespoon

Pepper and salt as desired

Method:

- Cucumbers are cut lengthwise, and the seeds are scooped out to provide a hollow hole for filling.

- Diced tomatoes, cucumbers, red onion, feta cheese crumbles, and chopped cilantro should all be combined in a bowl.

- Salt, pepper, parsley, lemon juice, olive oil, and ChatGPT. Blend well.

- Insert the Greek salad mixture into each hollowed-out half of the cucumber.

- As a light and energizing snack or starter, serve cold.

Guacamole and Veggie Sticks

Ingredients:

Two mature avocados

1 sliced small tomato

1/4 cup red onion, chopped

1/4 cup finely minced fresh cilantro

A teaspoon of lime juice

1 minced garlic clove

Pepper and salt as desired

A variety of vegetable sticks for dipping (carrot, celery, bell pepper)

Method:

- Remove the pits from the avocados, then scoop out the meat into a basin.
- With a fork, mash the avocado until it has the required consistency.
- To the mashed avocado, add diced tomato, red onion, cilantro, lime juice, minced garlic, salt, and pepper. To blend, thoroughly stir.

- To taste, adjust the spices.

- Serve the guacamole with a variety of
  veggie sticks for a wholesome and
  high-fiber snack.

These dishes provide alternatives that are low in
sodium, abundant in nutrients, and excellent for
those with diabetes and renal illness. They are
also made to be diabetic-friendly and
kidney-health sensitive.

Chapter Six

Refreshing Beverages for Diabetic Renal Health

Mint-Cucumber Infused Water

Ingredients:

One cucumber, thinly sliced Fresh mint leaves

Water

Method:

- In a pitcher, combine some fresh mint leaves with the cucumber slices.

- Add water to the pitcher.

- For at least two hours, let the ingredients soak in the refrigerator.

- For a cool and hydrating beverage, pour the cucumber-mint-infused water over ice.

Blended Berry-Basil

Ingredients:

1 cup of mixed berries

1 little banana

A few leaves of fresh basil

A single cup of unsweetened almond milk (or
your chosen milk alternative)

Ice cubes, if desired

Method:

- Blend the mixed berries, banana, basil
  leaves, almond milk, and frozen basil in
  a blender.

- Blend everything well until it's smooth.

- For a cold smoothie, you may add ice
  cubes.

- Enjoy the vivid flavors of this nourishing
  and kidney-friendly smoothie after
  pouring it into a glass.

Iced Tea with Lemon-Lime

Ingredients:

Brewed unsweetened green tea in two glasses

Lemon juice from one

1 lime's juice

To taste, use stevia or your chosen artificial

sweetener.

An ice cube

Method:

- Make the green tea, then let it cool.
- The chilled green tea should be mixed with the lime, lemon, and sweetener in a pitcher.
- To fully combine the flavors, stir well.
- Individual glasses should be filled with ice cubes before adding the lemon-lime iced tea.
- Enjoy this hydrating and refreshing beverage after adjusting the sweetness to your taste.

Watermelon-Cucumber

Ingredients:

2 cups of watermelon, chopped

1 lime juice and 1/2 a cucumber, chopped

Fresh mint leaves

Water

Method:

- Blend some fresh mint leaves, cucumber, watermelon, and lime juice.

- Blend everything well until it's smooth.

- If preferred, strain the mixture to get rid of any pulp.

- Ice cubes should be placed in glasses before adding the watermelon-cucumber combination.

- Enjoy this hydrated and cooling summer cooler with more fresh mint leaves as a garnish.

Iced Tea with Hibiscus

Ingredients:

2 cups of brewed, unsweetened hibiscus tea

Orange juice, to taste, with Stevia or your

choice of artificial sweetener

An ice cube

Method:

- Make the hibiscus tea, then let it cool.

- The chilled hibiscus tea, orange juice,
  and sweetener should all be combined in
  a pitcher.

- To fully combine the flavors, stir well.

- Hibiscus iced tea should be poured over
  individual glasses of iced tea after adding
  ice cubes.

- Enjoy this colorful, kidney-friendly iced
  tea after adjusting the sweetness to your
  liking.

Pineapple-Basil Lemonade

Ingredients:

1 cup of pieces of fresh pineapple

Two lemons' juice

A few leaves of fresh basil

To taste, use stevia or your chosen artificial

sweetener.

Water

An ice cube

Method:

- Blend the fresh pineapple chunks, lemon juice, basil leaves, sugar, and a little bit of water in a blender.
- Blend everything well until it's smooth.
- Add water to the combined mixture in a pitcher to thin it to the right consistency.

Chapter Seven

Diabetic Renal Desserts and Treats

Berry Chia Pudding

Ingredients:

Chia seeds, 1/4 cup

A single cup of unsweetened almond milk (or your chosen milk alternative)

One-half teaspoon of vanilla extract

To taste, use stevia or your chosen artificial sweetener.

For the topping, use fresh berries (strawberries, blueberries, and raspberries).

Method:

- Chia seeds, almond milk, vanilla extract, and sweetener should all be combined in a bowl.

- Stir everything together completely.

- The mixture should be chilled for at least two hours or overnight so that it may thicken and take on the consistency of pudding.

- Individual bowls or jars of chia pudding should be served with fresh berries on top.

Apple Slices Baked

Ingredients:

2 apples of medium size

1 teaspoon melted unsalted butter

1/8 teaspoon cinnamon powder

To taste, use stevia or your chosen artificial sweetener.

Method:

- A baking sheet should be lined with parchment paper and the oven should be preheated to 350°F (175°C).

- Apples should be cored and cut into thin rings.

- Sliced apples should be mixed with melted butter, cinnamon powder, and sugar in a bowl.

- On the prepared baking sheet, arrange the apple slices in a single layer.

- Bake the apples for 20 to 25 minutes, or until they are soft and just beginning to caramelize.

- Before serving the baked apple slices as a naturally sweet dessert, let them cool just a little.

Greek Yogurt Dessert

Ingredients:

1 cup of Greek yogurt, plain

1/4 cup chopped nuts (pistachios, almonds, or walnuts)

Fresh strawberries, blueberries, and raspberries make up 1/4 cup.

1 tbsp of optional sugar-free granola

To taste, use stevia or your chosen artificial sweetener.

Method:

- Greek yogurt, chopped almonds, fresh berries, and sugar-free granola should be arranged in a glass or dish.
- Till all the ingredients are utilized, keep layering.
- If desired, drizzle with a little sweetness.
- As a dessert or snack that is loaded with nutrients and protein, serve the Greek yogurt parfait cold.

Chocolate Avocado Mousse

Ingredients:

Two mature avocados

Unsweetened cocoa powder, 1/4 cup

(Or any other favorite milk alternative) 1/4 cup unsweetened almond milk

Vanilla extract, 1 teaspoon

To taste, use stevia or your chosen artificial sweetener.

Topping of fresh berries is optional.

Method:

- The avocados, cocoa powder, almond milk, vanilla extract, and sweetener should all be combined in a blender or food processor.
- Blend till creamy and smooth.
- If necessary, taste and adjust the sweetness.
- Pour the chocolate avocado mousse into serving bowls, then chill and set in the refrigerator for at least 30 minutes.
- Enjoy this decadent dessert, and if you want, garnish it with fresh berries.

Freeze Banana Bites

Ingredients:

Two ripe bananas

1/4 cup of unsweetened almond or peanut butter

(Optional) Shredded coconut without sugar

Method:

- Bananas should be peeled and chopped into bite-sized pieces.
- Each piece of banana should have a thin layer of almond or peanut butter spread on one side.
- Optional: For more texture and taste, roll the side of the banana chunk covered in peanut butter in the shredded coconut.
- On a baking sheet covered with parchment paper, arrange the banana bits.
- The banana bits should be frozen for at least two hours, or until they are solid.
- The banana bits should be placed in a freezer-safe container once they have frozen.

- Enjoy this delicious and filling delight of frozen banana pieces.

Coconut Chia Seed Popsicles

Ingredients:

1 can of unsweetened coconut milk (14 ounces).

Chia seeds, 2 teaspoons

To taste, use stevia or your chosen artificial sweetener.

Slices of fresh fruit may be used as a garnish.

Method:

- The coconut milk, chia seeds, and sweetener should all be combined in a dish.
- To make sure the chia seeds are dispersed equally, stir well.
- To enable the chia seeds to absorb the liquid, let the mixture rest for about 10 minutes.

- Using popsicle molds, pour the ingredients and, if preferred, top with fresh fruit pieces.

- Popsicle sticks should be put into the molds.

- Make sure the popsicles are thoroughly frozen by freezing them for at least 4-6 hours.

- Enjoy these creamy and cooling delights by removing the popsicles from the molds once they have frozen.

These diabetic renal sweets and snacks are created to be low in sugar, ideal for diabetics, and kidney-friendly.

Chapter Eight

Special Occasion Recipes for Diabetic Renal Diet

Aromatized Salmon

Ingredients:

4 filets of salmon

Olive oil, two teaspoons

2 minced garlic cloves

1 tablespoon freshly chopped dill and 2

tablespoons freshly chopped parsley

Pepper and salt as desired

Serving slices of lemon

Method:

- A baking sheet should be lined with parchment paper and the oven should be preheated to 400°F (200°C).
- Place and arrange the filets on a baking sheet

- Olive oil, minced garlic, chopped dill, chopped parsley, salt, and pepper should all be combined in a small dish.
- The salmon fillets should be evenly covered in the herb mixture.
- When the salmon is cooked through and flakes readily with a fork, bake for 12 to 15 minutes.
- Lemon wedges should be served with herb-roasted fish.

Lemon Herb Chicken on the Grill

Ingredients:

4 skinless, boneless breasts of chicken

Lemon juice from one

Olive oil, two teaspoons

2 minced garlic cloves

1 tablespoon freshly chopped rosemary

1 tablespoon of freshly chopped thyme

Pepper and salt as desired

Method:

- Lemon juice, olive oil, minced garlic, rosemary, thyme, salt, and pepper should all be combined in a bowl.

- Pour the marinade over the chicken breasts in a shallow dish, being sure to coat them completely.

- For at least 30 minutes, marinate the dish, cover it, and place it in the refrigerator.

- Set the grill's temperature to medium-high.

- Chicken breasts should be taken out of the marinade after shaking off any extra.

- The chicken should be cooked through after grilling for 6 to 8 minutes on each side.

- Before serving, let the chicken rest for a few minutes.

Bell Peppers Stuffed with Quinoa

Ingredients:

1 cup cooked quinoa and 1/2 cup sliced zucchini with 4 bell peppers (of any color), tops and seeds removed

1/2 cup yellow squash, diced

1/4 cup red onion, chopped

tomato dice, one-fourth cup

1/4 cup feta cheese crumbles

1 tablespoon freshly chopped basil

Pepper and salt as desired

Method:

- Prepare a baking dish and preheat the oven to 375°F (190°C).
- Cooked quinoa, diced yellow and zucchini squash, diced red onion, diced tomatoes, crumbled feta cheese, chopped basil, salt, and pepper should all be combined in a dish.

- Place the quinoa mixture into the bell
  peppers before placing them on the
  prepared baking dish.

- Bake the peppers for 25 to 30 minutes, or
  until they are soft and the filling is
  well-cooked.

- Before serving, take them out of the oven
  and allow them to cool somewhat.

Mushroom and Spinach Risotto

Ingredients:

Olive oil, 1 tbsp

1 cup sliced button mushrooms or cremini

2 minced garlic cloves

Arborio rice, 1 cup

Low-sodium chicken or veggie broth, 4 cups

Fresh spinach leaves, 1 cup

Grated Parmesan cheese, 1/4 cup

Add salt and pepper to taste.

Method:

- Over medium heat, put the olive oil in a large pan.

- Sauté the mushrooms until they are browned and softened after adding the sliced mushrooms and chopped garlic.

- Arborio rice should be added and continuously stirred for 1 to 2 minutes.

- Heat the broth to a hot temperature in a different saucepan over medium heat.

- Add the heated broth to the rice mixture gradually, approximately 1/2 cup at a time. Before adding extra broth, stir continuously until the liquid has been absorbed.

- For the next 20 to 25 minutes, add broth while stirring, until the rice is creamy and soft.

- Fresh spinach leaves should be added and cooked until wilted.

- Add the grated Parmesan cheese after turning off the heat in the skillet.

- Add pepper and salt to taste

- Before serving, let the risotto take a few
  minutes to rest.

Baked Eggplant Parmesan

Ingredients:

1 big eggplant, cut into rounds about 1/4 inch
thick.

1 cup low-sodium marinara sauce

1/2 cup part-skim mozzarella cheese, shredded

Grated Parmesan cheese, 1/4 cup

1/4 cup of whole wheat breadcrumbs

1 tablespoon freshly chopped basil

1 tablespoon freshly chopped parsley

Pepper and salt as desired

Method:

- Bake at 375°F (190°C) for 15 minutes
  using a baking sheet lined with
  parchment paper.

- Lay the eggplant slices out on the baking sheet, then sprinkle them with a little salt and pepper.

- The eggplant slices should be baked for 10 to 12 minutes, or until they are soft.

- Breadcrumbs, grated Parmesan cheese, chopped basil, and parsley should all be combined in a small basin.

- Each slice of eggplant should have a thin coating of marinara sauce on it.

- The breadcrumb mixture should be distributed evenly over the sauce.

- Sprinkle some shredded mozzarella cheese on top of each piece.

- When the cheese is melted and bubbling, put the baking sheet back in the oven and bake for a further 10-15 minutes.

- If preferred, add more fresh herbs as a garnish before serving.

Grilled Vegetable Skewers

Ingredients:

Sliced zucchini from 1

1 sliced yellow squash

One red bell pepper, chopped

One red onion, chopped

Eight cherry tomatoes

Olive oil, two teaspoons

1/4 cup balsamic vinegar

Italian seasoning, 1 teaspoon, of dry

Pepper and salt as desired

Method:

- Set the grill's temperature to medium.

- Sliced zucchini, yellow squash, bell pepper, red onion, and cherry tomatoes should be threaded onto skewers.

- Mix the olive oil, balsamic vinegar, dry Italian spice, salt, and pepper in a small bowl.

- Evenly coat the veggie skewers with the oil and vinegar mixture.

- The skewers should be cooked on the preheated grill for 10 to 12 minutes, turning them over once or twice, or until the veggies are soft and just beginning to brown.

- Before serving, take the skewers from the grill and let them cool slightly.

Chapter Nine

Cooking Techniques for Diabetic Renal Health

There are several methods you may use when cooking for diabetic renal health to make scrumptious and healthy meals while taking into account the dietary limits and recommendations for those with diabetes and kidney troubles. The following cooking methods may help diabetics maintain good kidney health:

Cooking on a grill is a well-liked technique that can be used to create savory and nutritious meals. Use skinless chicken, fish, lean beef, or hog slices as lean protein sources while grilling. Choose homemade marinades prepared with herbs, spices, and low-sodium ingredients instead of marinating meat in sweet or high-sodium sauces. Bell peppers, zucchini, and eggplant are just a few of the veggies that may be grilled to add taste and nutrition.

A moderate cooking method that helps preserve the food's natural aromas and nutrients is steaming. It works especially well with fish and veggies. Vegetables' brilliant colors and crisp texture are preserved during steaming, which reduces the need for additional fats or oils. Pick low-mercury fish to steam, such as tilapia, trout, or salmon, which are also high in omega-3 fatty acids.

Roasting or Baking is a flexible cooking method that enables you to produce delectable foods with no additional fat. To improve the flavor, use lean meats like chicken, turkey, or fish and marinate them in herbs, spices, and citrus juices. Additionally, you may roast veggies like cauliflower, Brussels sprouts, or sweet potatoes to bring out their inherent sweetness and make a filling side dish.

Stir-frying is the rapid, oil-free preparation of tiny amounts of food in a hot pan. By using this method, you may hasten the cooking process while preserving the foods' original tastes and textures. Use non-stick cookware and a little canola or olive oil or other heart-healthy oil while cooking. To make a balanced and delectable supper, fill your stir-fry with vibrant

veggies, lean proteins, and fragrant herbs and
spices.

Simmering food in liquid, such as water or
broth, is a mild cooking technique called
poaching. For fragile foods like fish or chicken
breasts, this method works nicely. Poaching
allows you to flavor food without adding too
much salt or fat. To improve the flavor of the
meal, add herbs, spices, and low-sodium broths.

The use of a variety of herbs and spices to
enhance the taste of your food rather than
depending just on salt and sugar. To give your
recipes more depth and complexity, try
combining ingredients such as garlic, ginger,
cumin, turmeric, thyme, rosemary, and basil.
Herbs and spices are a fantastic method to
enhance taste without using a lot of salt.

Make your dressings and sauces, store-bought
sauces and dressings often include undetectable
sugars, a lot of salt, and bad fats. Instead, use
handmade products created with high-quality
ingredients. To make tasty, low-sodium
dressings, use items like vinegar, herbs, and
spices, as well as lemon juice. Consider

preparing fresh tomato-based sauces or creamy sauces with low-fat dairy substitutes like Greek yogurt for sauces.

Portion control is crucial, even if cooking methods are very vital for the health of diabetic kidneys. Managing portion sizes reduces calorie consumption and helps control blood sugar levels. To make sure you are providing the proper quantities, use measuring cups, food scales, or portion control containers.

Chapter Ten

Conclusion

Being newly diagnosed with diabetes and kidney health issues may be difficult and stressful. But you can take this road and adopt a fit and content lifestyle if you have the correct information, resources, and assistance. This Diabetic Renal Diet Cookbook is a thorough resource and companion for those starting this new phase of their lives.

The basic tenets of a diabetic renal diet have been examined throughout this cookbook, offering helpful insights into the dietary requirements and concerns of those with diabetes and kidney problems. We have covered a broad variety of dishes, including appetizers, drinks, main meals, and desserts, all of which have been specifically designed to satisfy the nutritional needs of this special community.

In addition to putting nutrition first, the recipes in this cookbook also highlight different tastes and ingredients. Incorporating lean proteins, healthy fats, fiber-rich carbs, and a range of fruits and vegetables, we have emphasized the usage of whole, fresh foods. We work to support optimum health, blood sugar management, and renal function by emphasizing nutrient-dense components.

In addition, we've emphasized cooking methods that optimize taste while consuming the least amount of bad fats, too much salt, and added sugars. We have shown that healthy cooking is fun and tasty by using grilling, steaming, baking, stir-frying, poaching, and other culinary techniques.

We urge you to tackle this new chapter as you begin it with an optimistic outlook and an open heart. Adopting a diabetic renal diet is not about restriction; rather, it is about celebrating the benefits of providing your body with healthful, tasty, and balanced meals. You will come across a wide range of culinary options that cater to your health and well-being if you have the time, patience, and desire to experiment with new ingredients and tastes.

Keep in mind that this cookbook serves as a source of inspiration, knowledge, and empowerment in addition to being a compilation of recipes. It is a tool to assist you in moving in the direction of improved health. Make use of it as a starting point to explore, adjust, and produce unique dishes that suit your preferences and tastes.

Finally, we want to thank you from the bottom of our hearts for entrusting us with your health and culinary endeavors. We hope that the Diabetic Renal Diet Cookbook will become a dependable friend, giving you the information, motivation, and helpful advice you need to succeed on your newly diagnosed path.

I hope you have a long and healthy life filled with joy and delicious meals.

www.ingramcontent.com/pod-product-compliance
Lightning Source LLC
Chambersburg PA
CBHW050042260726
48658CB00005B/1724